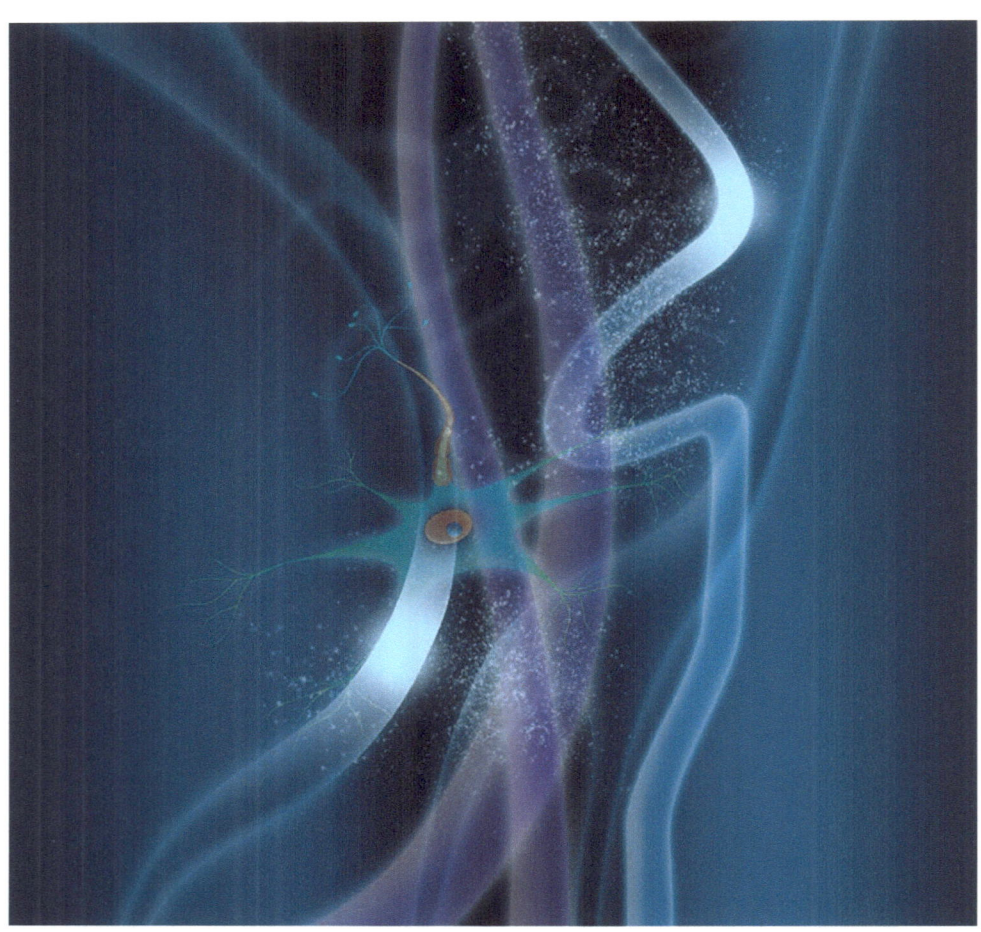

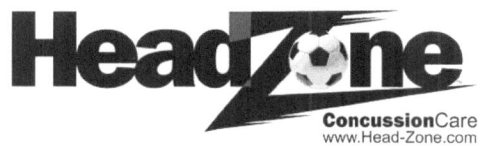

CLINICAL MANUAL FOR PEDIATRIC SPORTS SPECIFIC
"RETURN TO PLAY" PROTOCOLS

CONTRIBUTING AUTHORS AND REVIEWERS:

Karen Laugel, MD, FAAP

Amanda Jenks, ATC, CSCS

Megan Bromley, MHS, PA-C

Diana Reichbind, MPH, MHS, PA-C

Kelly Mitchell, BS Exercise Science

*Illustrations and layout by
Trevor Stone Irvin | IrvinProductions*

CLINICAL MANUAL FOR PEDIATRIC SPORTS SPECIFIC "RETURN TO PLAY" PROTOCOLS

The American Academy of Pediatrics supports adherence to a graduated "Return to Play" (RTP) protocol for children recovering from a concussion (1), as proposed by the International Conference on Concussion in Sport (ICCS) (2). In 2014, Keith May et al published pediatric RTP guidelines (3), which included sports specific exercises for the following nine protocols: cheerleading, baseball/softball, basketball, football, gymnastics, ice hockey, lacrosse, soccer, and wrestling.

Our regional pediatric ambulatory concussion care center (4) expanded upon these guidelines, adding sports specific instructions that include aerobic exercise, balance and strength, change of plane, and activities involving head rotation. In addition, we included a 'general activities' RTP protocol for children returning only to gym or recess, resistance training for those desiring gym workouts, and an additional fifteen sports for children, teens,
and young adults (see enclosed sports-specific protocols).

Our pediatric sport-specific RTP protocols can be used to determine readiness for return to play as per the ICCS, or can be used to create sub-symptom conditioning programs for those children who are still in recovery. For the latter group, we first administer a Buffalo Concussion Treadmill challenge test (5) adapted for pediatrics, to determine safe level of exercise (refer to HeadZone Pediatric Clinical Guide Series: Manual 2).

REFERENCES

1) Halstead ME, Walter KD; Clinical Report—Sport Related Concussion in Children and Adolescents. Pediatrics. 2010; 126 (3): 597-616
2) McCrory P, Meeuwisse W, Dvorak J, et al; Consensus statement on concussion in sport—the 5th international conference on concussion in sport held in Berlin, October 2016. Br J Sports Med. 2017; 0: 1-10
3) May KH, Marshall DL, Burns TG et al; Pediatric sports specific return to play guidelines following a concussion. International Journal of Sports Physical Therapy; 9 (2): 242-255
4) HeadZone LLC, Comprehensive Concussion Care Center, 2 Ivy Brook Road, Suite 213, Shelton, CT 06484
5) Leddy JJ, Willer B. Use of graded exercise testing in concussion and return-to-activity management. Curr Sports Med Rep. 2013; 12 (6): 370-376
6) Leddy JJ, Baker JG, Kozlowski K, Bisson L, Willer B. Reliability of a graded exercise test for assessing recovery from concussion. Clin J Sport Med. 2011;21(2):89-94
7) Leddy JJ, Baker JG, Haider MN, Hinds A, Willer B. A physiological approach to prolonged recovery from sport-related concussion. J Athl Train. 2017;52(3):299-308
8) Willer, Barry. "Evaluation of Exercise Tolerance." Brain Injury Alliance of Connecticut Annual Meeting. Hilton Hotel, Hartford. 17 March 2017. Lecture.
9) Malviya S, Voepel-Lewis T, Burke C. The revised FLACC observational pain tool: improved reliability and validity for pain assessment in children with cognitive impairment. Pediatric Anesthesia. 2006; 16: 258-265

GENERAL ACTIVITIES

If headache, dizziness, or any other symptoms occur during any phase, STOP exercising.
Wait 24 hours, and then resume activity at the previous symptom-free Phase/Day.
NOTE: Protective equipment should be worn when warranted (e.g., helmet, elbow & knee pads)

Exertion Phase	Cardio	Balance/Strength	P.E./Activities/Sports
Phase 1 At least 15-20 minutes	<ul><li>Walking outside with dog</li><li>Treadmill walking</li><li>Stationary bike</li><li>Arm Bike</li></ul>	<ul><li>Single leg balance (3 x 30 sec)</li><li>Tandem balance (one foot in front of the other 2 x 15 sec)</li><li>Neck exercises (see handout)</li></ul>	Examples:<ul><li>Stretching</li><li>Walking in P.E.</li><li>Mother May I</li><li>Bocce</li></ul>
Phase 2 20-30 minutes	<ul><li>Elliptical</li><li>Stationary bike</li><li>Swimming with kickboard</li><li>Stair master</li><li>Light jogging</li><li>Light jump rope</li></ul>	Perform **1 x 10** of the following:<ul><li>Plank (10 sec hold)</li><li>Leg lifts</li><li>Stationary lunge</li><li>Body-weight squat</li><li>Step-up onto stair/box,</li><li>Push-up</li></ul>-Yoga and Pilates class (limit head movement) -Continue balance exercises (above)	<ul><li>**Activities with NO risk of collision or contact.**</li><li>**NO activities with multiple balls flying through the air**</li></ul>Examples:<ul><li>Light throw and catch (nerf/ sponge ball)</li><li>Stationary dribble/shoot (Play 'horse')</li><li>Soccer footwork</li><li>'Marking' dance/cheer moves</li><li>Stick handling with puck on ground (not on ice)</li><li>Swing a bat/hit off a tee (Wiffle ball)</li><li>Mini-golf (putting)</li><li>Catching ground balls from knees</li><li>Bounce a tennis ball against wall</li><li>Hop-scotch</li><li>Marco Polo</li><li>Four Square</li></ul>
Phase 3 30-40 minutes	<ul><li>Running</li><li>Sprinting as tolerated</li><li>Accelerate to full speed with change of directions (cuts)</li><li>Swimming (start with breast stroke/ side stroke then freestyle, etc. if tolerated)</li></ul>	Continue above exercises; Add **2 x 10** of the following:<ul><li>Bicycle crunches</li><li>Plank with head rotation</li><li>Bear walk 10 feet</li><li>Crab walk 10 feet</li><li>Single-leg squat</li><li>Walking lunges and 3-way lunges</li><li>Jumping jacks</li><li>Squat and jump</li><li>Wall ball passes</li><li>Single-leg balance with forward reach to floor</li></ul>	<ul><li>Can incorporate light hand-touch contact only</li><li>**No competitive game play**</li><li>Wear contrast color jersey to indicate no collision</li></ul>Examples:<ul><li>Freeze tag (no pushing)</li><li>Soccer drills</li><li>Basketball drills</li><li>Badminton</li><li>Capture the flag</li><li>Tennis</li></ul>
Phase 4 40-60 minutes	<ul><li>Continue Phase 3 Cardio, increasing in duration</li></ul>	Continue above exercises; Add **3 x 10** of the following:<ul><li>Skip 10 ft.</li><li>Walking lunges and 3-way lunges with weight</li><li>Jump onto/off box</li><li>Squat and jump with direction change (forward/back; left/right)</li><li>Star jumps</li><li>Burpees</li><li>Mountain climbers</li></ul>	<ul><li>Can incorporate controlled contact</li></ul>Examples:<ul><li>Kickball</li><li>Volleyball</li><li>Baseball/Softball</li><li>Flag football</li></ul>
Phase 5 > 60 minutes	Full Activity	Full Activity	All competitive game play/Full P.E. Class/Full Activity

BASEBALL/SOFTBALL

If headache, dizziness, or any other symptoms occur during any Phase, STOP exercising, wait <u>24 hours</u>, and then resume activity at the <u>previous</u> symptom-free Phase/Day.
NOTE: Protective equipment should be worn when warranted (ex. helmet, elbow & knee pads)

Exertion Phase	Cardio	Balance/Strength	Sports Drills
Phase 1 At least 15-20 minutes	- Walking outside - Treadmill walking - Stationary bike - Arm Bike	- Single leg balance - Tandem balance (one foot in front of the other) - Neck exercises (see handout)	- Light stretching with team or in P.E class - May <u>walk</u> around gym, track, field in P.E. class
Phase 2 20 - 30 minutes	- Walking (speed walk, walk uphill) - Elliptical - Stairmaster - Swim with kickboard - Light jump rope - Light jogging	- Core exercises without head movement (ex. planks, leg lifts, etc.) - Body-weight exercises 1x10 (stationary lunges, squats, step-ups, push-ups, triceps dips, etc.) - Yoga and Pilates class (limit head movement) - Continue balance exercises	- Activities with NO risk of collision or contact - NO activities with multiple balls flying through the air Examples: - Light throw and catch - Swing a bat/hit off a tee (Wiffle ball) - Catching ground balls from knees
Phase 3 30 – 40 minutes	- Running & sprinting - Accelerate to full speed with change of directions (cuts) - Emphasize quick acceleration and deceleration	- Core exercises w/head movement (ex. bicycle crunches, Russian twists, plank with head rotation) - Low-weight, high-repetition exercises 3x10 (ex. single-leg squats, walking lunges, 3- way lunges, bicep curls, bench press, etc.) - Dynamic warm-up (jogging, high knees, butt kicks, lunges, hip rotations etc.) - Jumping/impact exercises (squat jumps, jumping jacks, wall ball passes, progress to box jumps) - Balance exercises (ex. single-leg balance with forward reach to floor)	- Agility/ladder drills - Base running drills w/no balls being hit - Fielding drills (ex. catching fly balls) - Pitchers – medium intensity throw and catch; progressing to game intensity - Pick off attempts (catcher – practice coming out of the crouch position) - Hit balls thrown lightly by coach; progress to hitting off pitching machine
Phase 4 40 – 60 minutes	- Continue Phase 3 cardio, increasing intensity duration	- Advanced core exercises (burpees, mountain climbers, etc.) - Can incorporate higher-weight, low-repetition exercises 4x3 (ex. Olympic Lifts, etc.) - Continue balance exercises	- Live batting practice (no live scrimmage) - Practice sliding (no live base running) - Practice diving for rolled balls from knees - Catchers can catch live batters
Phase 5 >60 minutes	Full contact practice participation	Full contact practice participation	Full contact practice participation

HeadZone www.Head-Zone.com

BASKETBALL

If headache, dizziness, or any other symptoms occur during any Phase, STOP exercising, wait <u>24 hours</u>, and then resume activity at the <u>previous</u> symptom-free Phase/Day.
(Updated September 2017)

Exertion Phase	Cardio	Balance/strength	Sports Drills
Phase 1 At least 15-20 minutes	- Walking outside - Treadmill walking - Stationary bike - Arm Bike	- Single leg balance - Tandem balance (one foot in front of the other) - Neck exercises (see handout)	- Light stretching with team or in P.E class - May <u>walk</u> around gym, track, field in P.E. class
Phase 2 20 - 30 minutes	- Walking (speed walk, walk uphill) - Elliptical - Stairmaster - Swim with kickboard - Light jump rope - Light jogging	- Core exercises without head movement (ex. planks, leg lifts, etc.) - Body-weight exercises 1x10 (stationary lunges, squats, step-ups, push-ups, triceps dips, etc.) - Yoga and Pilates class (limit head movement) - Continue balance exercises	- Activities with NO risk of collision or contact - NO activities with multiple balls flying through the air Examples: - Light passing drills - Stationary dribbling - Stationary shooting - Play 'horse' - Practice foul shots - NO standing under basket getting rebounds
Phase 3 30 – 40 minutes	- Running & sprinting - Accelerate to full speed with change of directions - Suicides	- Core exercises w/head movement (ex. bicycle crunches, Russian twists, plank with head rotation) - Low-weight, high-repetition exercises 3x10 (ex. single-leg squats, walking lunges, 3-way lunges, bicep curls, bench press, etc.) - Dynamic warm-up (jogging, high skips, side shuffles, jumping jacks, high knees, butt kicks, etc.) - Jumping/impact exercises (squat jumps, jumping jacks, lateral hops, wall ball passes, box jumps) - Balance exercises (ex. single-leg balance with forward reach to floor)	All drills with **NO OPPONENT** and **NO** chance of collision with another player - Agility/ladder drills - Shooting drills - Full court team passing drills (3-man weave, partner pass) - Team drills with no opponent (ex. offensive drill vs. no defense) - Solo rebounding (no opponent)
Phase 4 40 – 60 minutes	- Continue Phase 3 Cardio, increasing in duration	- Advanced core exercises (burpees, mountain climbers, etc.) - Can incorporate higher-weight, low-repetition exercises 4x3 (ex. Olympic Lifts, etc.) - Continue balance exercises	**Incorporate drills with an opponent (no live scrimmaging)** - Offense vs. defense drills - Individual drills (1 v 1, 2 v 1, 3 v 2) - Post moves and rebounding with assisted pad contact (progress to player contact)
Phase 5 >60 minutes	Full contact practice participation	Full contact practice participation	Full contact practice participation

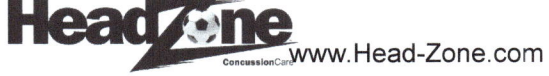
www.Head-Zone.com

CHEERLEADING

If headache, dizziness, or any other symptoms occur during any Phase, STOP exercising, wait <u>24 hours</u>, and then resume activity at the <u>previous</u> symptom-free Phase/Day.

Exertion Phase	Cardio	Balance/Strength	Sports Drills
Phase 1 At least 15-20 minutes	- Walking outside - Treadmill walking - Stationary bike - Arm Bike	- Single leg balance - Tandem balance (one foot in front of the other) - Neck exercises (see handout)	- Light stretching with team or in P.E class - May <u>walk</u> around gym, track, field in P.E. class
Phase 2 20 - 30 minutes	- Walking (speed walk, walk uphill) - Elliptical - Stairmaster - Swim with kickboard - Light jump rope - Light jogging	- Core exercises without head movement (ex. planks, leg lifts, etc.) - Body-weight exercises 1x10 (stationary lunges, squats, step-ups, push-ups, triceps dips, etc.) - Yoga and Pilates class (limit head movement) - Continue balance exercises	- Activities with NO risk of collision or contact - NO activities with multiple balls flying through the air Examples: - Practice cheers (practice in a low-volume area if sensitive to noise) - 'Marking' dance moves, stunt routine, and tumbling
Phase 3 30 – 40 minutes	- Running & sprinting - Accelerate to full speed with change of directions (cuts) - Emphasize quick acceleration and deceleration	- Core exercises w/head movement (ex. bicycle crunches, Russian twists, plank with head rotation) - Low-weight, high-repetition exercises 3x10 (ex. single-leg squats, walking lunges, 3-way lunges, bicep curls, bench press, etc.) - Dynamic warm-up (jogging, high knees, butt kicks, lunges, hip rotations etc.) - Jumping/impact exercises (squat jumps, jumping jacks, wall ball passes, progress to box jumps) - Balance exercises (ex. single-leg balance with forward reach to floor)	**NO stunting or running tumbling at this phase** May begin the following: - Jumps (toe-touch, Herkie, etc.) - 15 yd. sprints (as in a tumbling pass) - Non-consecutive stationary tumbling (cartwheel, round-off, walkover, forward roll, single handspring) - Can do dance/cheer portion of competition routine (no rapid head movements or moves where head could hit the floor) - Mark stunt portion of routine
Phase 4 40 – 60 minutes	- Continue Phase 3 cardio, increasing intensity and duration	- Advanced core exercises (burpees, mountain climbers, etc.) - Can incorporate higher-weight, lower-repetition exercises - Continue balance exercises	**May practice running tumbling and stunting but not in competition routine run-through** May begin the following: - Running tumbling passes (single flip progressing to multiple as tolerated) - <u>Stunt progression</u>: begin with double-leg stunts advancing to single-leg stunts USING EXTRA SPOTTERS - Cradle catch (no spins) - <u>Basket tosses</u>: start with low-level tosses progressing to higher-level tosses with spins USING EXTRA SPOTTERS
Phase 5 >60 minutes	Full practice participation	Full practice participation	- Full practice participation (limit number of full competition run-throughs) - **No cheering or performing at games until clearance by your health care professional**

HeadZone www.Head-Zone.com

COLOR GUARD

If headache, dizziness, or any other symptoms occur during any Phase, STOP exercising, wait <u>24 hours</u>, and then resume activity at the <u>previous</u> symptom-free Phase/Day.

Exertion Phase	Cardio	Balance/Strength	Sports Drills
Phase 1 At least 15-20 minutes	- Walking outside - Treadmill walking - Stationary bike - Arm Bike	- Single leg balance - Tandem balance (one foot in front of the other) - Neck exercises (see handout)	- Light stretching with team or in P.E class - May <u>walk</u> around gym, track, field in P.E. class
Phase 2 20 - 30 minutes	- Walking (speed walk, walk uphill) - Elliptical - Stairmaster - Swim with kickboard - Light jump rope - Light jogging	- Core exercises without head movement (ex. planks, leg lifts, etc.) - Body-weight exercises 1x10 (stationary lunges, squats, step-ups, push-ups, triceps dips, etc.) - Yoga and Pilates class (limit head movement) - Continue balance exercises	- Activities with NO risk of collision or contact - NO activities with multiple balls flying through the air Examples: - 'Marking' dance/flag moves - NO tosses
Phase 3 30 – 40 minutes	- Maximize aerobic activity - Include running & sprinting - Accelerate to full speed with change of directions (cuts)	- Core exercises w/head movement (ex. bicycle crunches, Russian twists, plank with head rotation) - Low-weight, high-repetition exercises 3x10 (ex. single-leg squats, walking lunges, 3- way lunges, bicep curls, bench press, etc.) - Dynamic warm-up (jogging, high knees, butt kicks, lunges, hip rotations etc.) - Jumping/impact exercises (squat jumps, jumping jacks, wall ball passes, progress to box jumps) - Balance exercises (ex. single-leg balance with forward reach to floor)	- Warm-up drills (spinning and technique exercises) - Dance warm-up drills - Flag work/weapon work on sidelines - No tosses
Phase 4 40 – 60 minutes	- Continue Phase 3 Cardio, increasing in duration	- Advanced core exercises (burpees, mountain climbers, etc.) - Can incorporate higher-weight, lower-repetition exercises - Continue balance exercises	- All warm-up drills (dance, etc.) - No OVERHEAD tosses - Half-run through of performance
Phase 5 >60 minutes	Full practice participation	Full practice participation	Full practice participation

HeadZone
www.Head-Zone.com

DANCE

If headache, dizziness, or any other symptoms occur during any Phase, STOP exercising, wait <u>24 hours</u>, and then resume activity at the <u>previous</u> symptom-free Phase/Day.

Exertion Phase	Cardio	Balance/Strength	Sports Drills
Phase 1 At least 15-20 minutes	<ul><li>Walking outside</li><li>Treadmill walking</li><li>Stationary bike</li><li>Arm Bike</li></ul>	<ul><li>Single leg balance</li><li>Tandem balance (one foot in front of the other)</li><li>Neck exercises (see handout)</li></ul>	<ul><li>Light stretching with team or in P.E class</li><li>May <u>walk</u> around gym, track, field in P.E. class</li></ul>
Phase 2 20 - 30 minutes	<ul><li>Walking (speed walk, walk uphill)</li><li>Elliptical</li><li>Stairmaster</li><li>Swim with kickboard</li><li>Light jump rope</li><li>Light jogging</li></ul>	<ul><li>Core exercises without head movement (ex. planks, leg lifts, etc.)</li><li>Body-weight exercises 1x10 (stationary lunges, squats, step-ups, push-ups, triceps dips, etc.)</li><li>Yoga and Pilates class (limit head movement)</li><li>Continue balance exercises</li></ul>	<ul><li>Activities with NO risk of collision or contact</li><li>NO activities with multiple balls flying through the air</li></ul>Examples:<ul><li>'Marking' dance moves</li><li>Stretching to maintain flexibility</li></ul>
Phase 3 30 – 40 minutes	<ul><li>Maximize aerobic activity</li><li>Include running & sprinting</li><li>Focus on accelerate and decelerate when running</li></ul>	<ul><li>Core exercises w/head movement (ex. bicycle crunches, Russian twists, plank with head rotation)</li><li>Low-weight, high-repetition exercises 3x10 (ex. single-leg squats, walking lunges, 3-way lunges, bicep curls, bench press, etc.)</li><li>Dynamic warm-up (jogging, high knees, butt kicks, lunges, hip rotations etc.)</li><li>Jumping/impact exercises (squat jumps, jumping jacks, wall ball passes, progress to box jumps)</li><li>Balance exercises (ex. single-leg balance with forward reach to floor)</li></ul>	-May participate in moderate intensity classes (ballet, jazz, contemporary, and tap classes) -Avoid any head contact with ground Limit the following:<ul><li>Turns: no more than 2 revolutions</li><li>Leaps: nothing that involves rapid head movement</li><li>Routines: limit number of run-throughs and mark moves that involve rapid head movement</li></ul>
Phase 4 40 – 60 minutes	<ul><li>Continue Phase 3 Cardio, increasing in duration</li></ul>	<ul><li>Advanced core exercises (burpees, mountain climbers, etc.)</li><li>Can incorporate higher-weight, lower-repetition exercises</li><li>Continue balance exercises</li></ul>	May participate in higher intensity classes (hip-hop, acro, jazz) May progress to:<ul><li>Full turns in routine</li><li>Full leaps in routine</li></ul>-Limit number of acro elements (avoid anything inverted)
Phase 5 >60 minutes	Full dance participation	Full dance participation	Full dance participation

HeadZone www.Head-Zone.com

DIVING

If headache, dizziness, or any other symptoms occur during any Phase, STOP exercising, wait <u>24 hours</u>, and then resume activity at the <u>previous</u> symptom-free Phase/Day.

Exertion Phase	Cardio	Balance/Strength	Sports Drills
Phase 1 At least 15-20 minutes	<ul><li>Walking outside</li><li>Treadmill walking</li><li>Stationary bike</li><li>Arm Bike</li></ul>	<ul><li>Single leg balance</li><li>Tandem balance (one foot in front of the other)</li><li>Neck exercises (see handout)</li></ul>	<ul><li>Light stretching with team or in P.E class</li><li>May <u>walk</u> around gym, track, field in P.E. class</li></ul>
Phase 2 20 - 30 minutes	<ul><li>Walking (speed walk, walk uphill)</li><li>Elliptical</li><li>Stairmaster</li><li>Swim with a kickboard</li><li>Light jump rope</li><li>Light jogging</li></ul>	<ul><li>Core exercises without head movement (ex. planks, leg lifts, etc.)</li><li>Body-weight exercises 1x10 (stationary lunges, squats, step-ups, push-ups, triceps dips, etc.)</li><li>Yoga and Pilates class (limit head movement)</li><li>Continue balance exercises</li></ul>	<ul><li>Activities with NO risk of collision or contact</li><li>NO activities with multiple balls flying through the air</li><li>Stretch to maintain flexibility</li></ul>
Phase 3 30 – 40 minutes	<ul><li>Maximize aerobic activity</li><li>Include running & sprinting</li><li>Accelerate to full speed with change of directions (cuts)</li></ul>	<ul><li>Core exercises w/head movement (ex. bicycle crunches, Russian twists, plank with head rotation)</li><li>Low-weight, high-repetition exercises 3x10 (ex. single-leg squats, walking lunges, 3- way lunges, bicep curls, bench press, etc.)</li><li>Dynamic warm-up (jogging, high knees, butt kicks, lunges, hip rotations etc.)</li><li>Jumping/impact exercises (squat jumps, jumping jacks, wall ball passes, progress to box jumps)</li><li>Balance exercises (ex. single-leg balance with forward reach to floor)</li></ul>	NO diving head first into pool from any height at this phase <ul><li>May jump feet first into pool</li><li>May practice handstands or cartwheels on dry land</li><li>Forward and backward rolls/flips while in the water</li><li>If available, may use trampoline <u>with safety belt</u> to practice dives</li><li>May practicing bouncing on the 1m board & jumping feet first into the pool</li></ul>
Phase 4 40-60 minutes	<ul><li>Continue Phase 3 Cardio, increasing in duration</li></ul>	<ul><li>Advanced core exercises (burpees, mountain climbers, etc.)</li><li>Can incorporate higher-weight, low-repetition exercises</li><li>Continue balance exercises</li></ul>	<ul><li>Start with forward dive into the water from the side of the pool</li><li>Progress to forward dives from 1m board only (begin with stationary dive then with bouncing)</li><li>Start with non-rotational dives (forward/backward etc. with tucks, pikes etc.)</li><li>Progress to twisting dives</li><li>Advance dive complexity gradually as tolerated</li></ul>
Phase 5 >60 minutes	Full practice participation	Full practice participation	<ul><li>Progress to 3m board following the same progression for the 1m board in Phase 4.</li><li>Consult with your clinician about resuming platform diving after you have resumed full activities on the 1 & 3m boards (if applicable)</li></ul>

HeadZone www.Head-Zone.com

EQUESTRIAN

If headache, dizziness, or any other symptoms occur during any Phase, STOP exercising, wait <u>24 hours</u>, and then resume activity at the <u>previous</u> symptom-free Phase/Day.
NOTE: Protective equipment should be worn when warranted (ex. helmet)

Exertion Phase	Cardio	Balance/Strength	Sports Drills
Phase 1 At least 15-20 minutes	<ul><li>Walking outside</li><li>Treadmill walking</li><li>Stationary bike</li><li>Arm Bike</li></ul>	<ul><li>Single leg balance</li><li>Tandem balance (one foot in front of the other)</li><li>Neck exercises (see handout)</li></ul>	<ul><li>Light stretching with team or in P.E class</li><li>May <u>walk</u> around gym, track, field in P.E. class</li></ul>
Phase 2 20 - 30 minutes	<ul><li>Walking (speed walk, walk uphill)</li><li>Elliptical</li><li>Stairmaster</li><li>Swim with kickboard</li><li>Light jump rope</li><li>Light jogging</li></ul>	<ul><li>Core exercises without head movement (ex. planks, leg lifts, etc.)</li><li>Body-weight exercises 1x10 (stationary lunges, squats, step-ups, push-ups, triceps dips, etc.)</li><li>Yoga and Pilates class (limit head movement)</li><li>Continue balance exercises</li></ul>	<ul><li>Activities with NO risk of collision or contact</li><li>NO activities with multiple balls flying through the air</li><li>Ride horse walking in ring</li></ul>
Phase 3 30 – 40 minutes	<ul><li>Maximize aerobic activity</li><li>Include running & sprinting</li><li>Accelerate to full speed with change of directions (cuts)</li></ul>	<ul><li>Core exercises w/head movement (ex. bicycle crunches, Russian twists, plank with head rotation)</li><li>Low-weight, high-repetition exercises 3x10 (ex. single-leg squats, walking lunges, 3- way lunges, bicep curls, bench press, etc.)</li><li>Dynamic warm-up (jogging, high knees, butt kicks, lunges, hip rotations etc.)</li><li>Jumping/impact exercises (squat jumps, jumping jacks, wall ball passes, progress to box jumps)</li><li>Balance exercises (ex. single-leg balance with forward reach to floor)</li></ul>	<ul><li>Trot with post progressing to light cantering</li><li>Short trail rides</li><li>Small jumps</li></ul>
Phase 4 40 – 60 minutes	<ul><li>Continue Phase 3 Cardio, increasing in duration</li></ul>	<ul><li>Advanced core exercises (burpees, mountain climbers, etc.)</li><li>Can incorporate higher-weight, low-repetition exercises</li><li>Continue balance exercises</li></ul>	<ul><li>Full cantering, progressing to gallop</li><li>Medium to large sized jumps</li><li>Long trail rides</li></ul>
Phase 5 >60 minutes	Full participation in practice/lessons	Full participation in practice/lessons	Full participation in practice/lessons

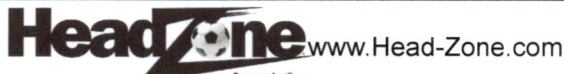
www.Head-Zone.com

FIELD HOCKEY

If headache, dizziness, or any other symptoms occur during any Phase, STOP exercising, wait <u>24 hours</u>, and then resume activity at the <u>previous</u> symptom-free Phase/Day.
NOTE: Protective equipment should be worn when warranted

Exertion Phase	Cardio	Balance/Strength	Sports Drills
Phase 1 At least 15-20 minutes	- Walking outside - Treadmill walking - Stationary bike - Arm Bike	- Single leg balance - Tandem balance (one foot in front of the other) - Neck exercises (see handout)	- Light stretching with team or in P.E class - May <u>walk</u> around gym, track, field in P.E. class
Phase 2 20 - 30 minutes	- Walking (speed walk, walk uphill) - Elliptical - Stairmaster - Swim with kickboard - Light jump rope - Light jogging	- Core exercises without head movement (ex. planks, leg lifts, etc.) - Body-weight exercises 1x10 (stationary lunges, squats, step-ups, push-ups, triceps dips, etc.) - Yoga and Pilates class (limit head movement) - Continue balance exercises	- Activities with NO risk of collision or contact - NO activities with multiple balls flying through the air Examples: - Low-intensity stick handling with a softer ball (not a field hockey ball)
Phase 3 30 – 40 minutes	- Running & sprinting - Accelerate to full speed with change of directions (cuts) - Emphasize quick acceleration and deceleration	- Core exercises w/head movement (ex. bicycle crunches, Russian twists, plank with head rotation) - Low-weight, high-repetition exercises 3x10 (ex. single-leg squats, walking lunges, 3- way lunges, bicep curls, bench press, etc.) - Dynamic warm-up (jogging, high knees, butt kicks, lunges, hip rotations etc.) - Jumping/impact exercises (squat jumps, jumping jacks, wall ball passes, progress to box jumps) - Balance exercises (ex. single-leg balance with forward reach to floor)	**Emphasize stick/ball handling drills without an opponent** Examples: - Agility/ladder drills - Footwork drills - Stick handling through cones as fast as you can - Short and long passing drills with coach, progressing to passing with teammates - Dragging the ball (be careful not to flick the ball) - Practice shooting (on own) - Run through plays without defense (i.e. corner drills)
Phase 4 40 – 60 minutes	- Continue Phase 3 cardio, increasing in intensity and duration	- Advanced core exercises (burpees, mountain climbers, etc.) - Can incorporate higher-weight, low-repetition exercises - Continue balance exercises	**Incorporate drills with an opponent (no live scrimmaging)** - Cone drills with opponent (get ball to your cone using stick skills) - Run through plays with defense (i.e. corner drills) - 1 v 1, 2 v 2, etc. - Blocking drills with ball - Shooting drills with team
Phase 5 >60 minutes	Full contact practice participation	Full contact practice participation	Full contact practice participation

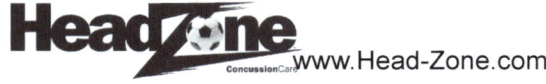
www.Head-Zone.com

FIGURE SKATING

If headache, dizziness, or any other symptoms occur during any Phase, STOP exercising, wait <u>24 hours</u>, and then resume activity at the <u>previous</u> symptom-free Phase/Day.
NOTE: Protective equipment should be worn when warranted

Exertion Phase	Cardio	Balance/Strength	Sports Drills
Phase 1 At least 15-20 minutes	<ul><li>Walking outside</li><li>Treadmill walking</li><li>Stationary bike</li><li>Arm Bike</li></ul>	<ul><li>Single leg balance</li><li>Tandem balance (one foot in front of the other)</li><li>Neck exercises (see handout)</li></ul>	<ul><li>Light stretching</li><li>May <u>walk</u> around gym, track, field in P.E. class</li></ul>
Phase 2 20 - 30 minutes	<ul><li>**NO ice skating**</li><li>Walking (speed walk, walk uphill)</li><li>Elliptical</li><li>Stairmaster</li><li>Swim with kickboard</li><li>Light jump rope</li><li>Light jogging</li></ul>	<ul><li>Core exercises without head movement (ex. planks, leg lifts, etc.)</li><li>Body-weight exercises 1x10 (stationary lunges, squats, step-ups, push-ups, triceps dips, etc.)</li><li>Yoga and Pilates class (limit head movement)</li><li>Continue balance exercises</li></ul>	<ul><li>Activities with NO risk of collision or contact</li><li>NO activities with multiple balls flying through the air</li></ul>Examples:<ul><li>Slide-board in PT</li><li>Mark choreography (OFF-ice)</li></ul>
Phase 3 30 – 40 minutes	Advanced **OFF-ice** cardio:<ul><li>Running & sprinting</li><li>Accelerate to full speed with change of directions (cuts)</li><li>Emphasize quick stops/ starts</li></ul>	<ul><li>Core exercises w/head movement (ex. bicycle crunches, Russian twists, plank with head rotation)</li><li>Low-weight, high-repetition exercises 3x10 (ex. single-leg squats, walking lunges, 3-way lunges, bicep curls, bench press, etc.)</li><li>Dynamic warm-up (jogging, high knees, butt kicks, lunges, hip rotations etc.)</li><li>Jumping/impact exercises (squat jumps, jumping jacks, wall ball passes, progress to box jumps)</li><li>Balance exercises (ex. single-leg balance with forward reach to floor)</li></ul>	*Progress to **ON-ice** drills:<ul><li>On/ off ice warm-up drills</li><li>Initiate skating</li><li>Forward and backward stroking with limited turns and twisting</li><li>No spins or jumps</li><li>Execute choreography (with or without music) with turns but with no spins or jumps</li></ul>
Phase 4 40 – 60 minutes	<ul><li>Continue Phase 3 Cardio, increasing in intensity and duration</li></ul>	<ul><li>Advanced core exercises (burpees, mountain climbers, etc.)</li><li>Higher-weight, low-repetition exercises 4x3 (ex. Olympic Lifts, etc.)</li><li>Continue balance exercises</li></ul>	<ul><li>Continue above exercises</li><li>*Basic spins and single jumps advancing to double jumps (if tolerated)</li></ul>
Phase 5 >60 minutes	Full practice	Full practice	Full participation including all spins and triple jumps

*Reference: U.S. Figure Skating, www.usfsa.org

HeadZone www.Head-Zone.com

FOOTBALL

If headache, dizziness, or any other symptoms occur during any Phase, STOP exercising, wait <u>24 hours</u>, and then resume activity at the <u>previous</u> symptom-free Phase/Day.
NOTE: Protective equipment should be worn when warranted (e.g., helmet, mouth guard, pads)

Exertion Phase	Cardio	Balance/Strength	Sports Drills
Phase 1 At least 15-20 minutes	- Walking outside - Treadmill walking - Stationary bike - Arm Bike	- Single leg balance - Tandem balance (one foot in front of the other) - Neck exercises (see handout)	- Light stretching with team or in P.E class - May <u>walk</u> around gym, track, field in P.E. class
Phase 2 20 - 30 minutes	- Walking (speed walk, walk uphill) - Elliptical - Stairmaster - Swim with a kickboard - Light jump rope - Light jogging	- Core exercises without head movement (ex. planks, leg lifts, etc.) - Body-weight exercises 1x10 (stationary lunges, squats, step-ups, push-ups, triceps dips, etc.) - Yoga and Pilates class (limit head movement) - Continue balance exercises (above)	- Activities with NO risk of collision or contact - NO activities with multiple balls flying through the air Examples: - Low-intensity throw and catch
Phase 3 30 – 40 minutes **Yellow (or contrast color) jersey should be worn to indicate NO contact** **Helmet ONLY, No pads**	- Running & sprinting - Accelerate to full speed with change of directions (cuts) - Emphasize quick acceleration and deceleration	- Core exercises w/head movement (ex. bicycle crunches, Russian twists, plank with head rotation) - Low-weight, high-repetition exercises 3x10 (ex. single-leg squats, walking lunges, 3-way lunges, bicep curls, bench press, etc.) - Dynamic warm-up (jogging, high knees, butt kicks, lunges, hip rotations etc.) - Jumping/impact exercises (squat jumps, jumping jacks, wall ball passes, progress to box jumps) - Balance exercises (ex. single-leg balance with forward reach to floor)	**Phase 3 is NON-CONTACT** Only <u>light hand-touch contact</u> in drills with NO chance of collision with another player - Agility/ladder drills - <u>Linemen/linebackers</u>: may do drills with light hand-touch contact only - <u>Quarterbacks</u>: un-opposed short and long passes progressing to competition intensity - <u>Skill players</u>: start with running routes un-opposed; progress to catching/defending passes with light hand-touch contact only - <u>Kickers/punters</u>: punting drills and medium range kicks (nothing live) - <u>Snapper</u>: few snaps (limit 10-15 per practice); no live snaps - No offense vs. defense drills
Phase 4 40 – 60 minutes **Full pads**	- Continue Phase 3 cardio, increasing in intensity and duration	- Advanced core exercises (burpees, mountain climbers, etc.) - Higher-weight, low-repetition exercises 4x3 (ex. Olympic Lifts, etc.) - Continue balance exercises (above)	Can initiate body contact and tackling in drills (no live scrimmage) - 1 v 1, 2 v 2, etc. - Offense vs. defense drills Tackle Progression: - Start with low-intensity hit/push of pads - Progress to sled push (full-intensity) then body contact/tackling in drills *HeadZone does not recommend tackling under high school age*
Phase 5 >60 minutes **Full pads**	Full contact practice participation	Full contact practice participation	Full contact practice/in-team scrimmage (no opposing team competitive scrimmage)

HeadZone www.Head-Zone.com

GYMNASTICS

If headache, dizziness, or any other symptoms occur during any Phase, STOP exercising, wait <u>24 hours</u>, and then resume activity at the <u>previous</u> symptom-free Phase/Day.

Exertion Phase	Cardio	Balance/Strength	Sports Drills
Phase 1 At least 15-20 minutes	- Walking outside - Treadmill walking - Stationary bike - Arm Bike	- Single leg balance - Tandem balance (one foot in front of the other) - Neck exercises (see handout)	- Light stretching with team or in P.E class - May <u>walk</u> around gym, track, field in P.E. class
Phase 2 20 - 30 minutes	- Walking (speed walk, walk uphill) - Elliptical - Stairmaster - Swim with kickboard - Light jump rope - Light jogging	- Core exercises without head movement (ex. planks, leg lifts, etc.) - Body-weight exercises 1x10 (stationary lunges, squats, step-ups, push-ups, triceps dips, etc.) - Yoga and Pilates class (limit head movement) - Continue balance exercises (above)	- Activities with NO risk of collision or contact - NO activities with multiple balls flying through the air Examples: - 'Marking' routines - Stretching to maintain flexibility
Phase 3 30 – 40 minutes	- Maximize aerobic activity - Include running & sprinting - Accelerate to full speed with change of directions (cuts)	- Core exercises w/head movement (ex. bicycle crunches, Russian twists, plank with head rotation) - Low-weight, high-repetition exercises 3x10 (ex. single-leg squats, walking lunges, 3- way lunges, bicep curls, bench press, etc.) - Dynamic warm-up (jogging, high knees, butt kicks, lunges, hip rotations etc.) - Jumping/impact exercises (squat jumps, jumping jacks, wall ball passes) - Single-leg and tandem balance on low beam (20 sec. hold) - Single-leg balance with forward reach to floor	- **Floor:** floor routine without running tumbling (progress to incorporating jumps, spins, turns); may try stationary beginner tumbling (handstand, cartwheel, bridge kick-overs, walkover, forward/backward roll) - **Beam:** choreography on low beam only; progress to jumps; no tumbling i.e. handspring, cartwheel, etc. on beam - **Bars:** swings on bars; higher level gymnasts can cast up to horizontal - **Vault:** run and jump off spring board (no vault)
Phase 4 40 – 60 minutes	- Continue Phase 3 Cardio, increasing in duration	- Advanced core exercises (burpees, mountain climbers, etc.) - Can incorporate higher-weight, lower-repetition exercises - Continue balance exercises	**Increase use of spotters (i.e beam, bars)** - **Floor:** Practice tumbling on tumble track, then progress to floor (single flip progressing to multiple as tolerated) - **Beam:** incorporate handsprings, etc. on low beam, progress to high beam - **Bars:** higher level gymnasts progress to kips, clear hips, stalder, giants, etc. on bars; start with no releases then progress to competition level - **Vault:** begin with level 1-2 vault and progress to competition level
Phase 5 >60 minutes	Full practice participation	Full practice participation	Full practice participation

HeadZone www.Head-Zone.com

ICE HOCKEY

If headache, dizziness, or any other symptoms occur during any Phase, STOP exercising, wait 24 hours, and then resume activity at the previous symptom-free Phase/Day.
NOTE: Protective equipment should be worn when warranted

Exertion Phase	Cardio	Balance/Strength	Sports Drills
Phase 1 At least 15-20 minutes	- Walking outside - Treadmill walking - Stationary bike - Arm Bike	- Single leg balance - Tandem balance (one foot in front of the other) - Neck exercises (see handout)	- Light stretching with team or in P.E class - May walk around gym, track, field in P.E. class
Phase 2 20 - 30 minutes	- **NO ice skating** - Walking (speed walk, walk uphill) - Elliptical - Stairmaster - Swim with kickboard - Light jump rope - Light jogging	- Core exercises without head movement (ex. planks, leg lifts, etc.) - Body-weight exercises 1x10 (stationary lunges, squats, step-ups, push-ups, triceps dips, etc.) - Yoga and Pilates class (limit head movement) - Continue balance exercises	- Activities with NO risk of collision or contact - NO activities with multiple balls flying through the air Examples: - Stick handling and low-intensity shooting/passing on ground (not on ice) - Slide-board in PT
Phase 3 30 – 40 minutes **Yellow (or contrast color) jersey should be worn to indicate NO contact** **Full pads**	Advanced **OFF-ice** cardio: - Running & sprinting - Accelerate to full speed with change of directions (cuts) - Emphasize quick stops/ starts Progress to **ON-ice** cardio: - Initiate skating - Progress to backward/lateral skating and sprinting with stick/puck handling	- Core exercises w/head movement (ex. bicycle crunches, Russian twists, plank with head rotation) - Low-weight, high-repetition exercises 3x10 (ex. single-leg squats, walking lunges, 3-way lunges, bicep curls, bench press, etc.) - Dynamic warm-up (jogging, high knees, butt kicks, lunges, hip rotations etc.) - Jumping/impact exercises (squat jumps, jumping jacks, wall ball passes, progress to box jumps) - Balance exercises (ex. single-leg balance with forward reach to floor)	-All drills with **NO OPPONENT** and **NO** chance of collision with another player - On/ off ice warm-up drills - Agility drills (i.e. Stick/puck handling, shooting, and passing) - Ladder agility drills Goaltenders: - Non-competitive goalie drills i.e. agility drills with tennis ball, block shots from coach (no rapid fire & no live scrimmage shots) - Work on movement required when puck is behind/in front of goal, and being passed from side to side
Phase 4 40 – 60 minutes **Full pads**	- Continue Phase 3 Cardio, increasing in intensity and duration	- Advanced core exercises (burpees, mountain climbers, etc.) - Higher-weight, low-repetition exercises 4x3 (ex. Olympic Lifts, etc.) - Continue balance exercises	**Incorporate drills with an opponent (no live scrimmaging)** - 1 v1, 2 v 2, etc. opponent drills (no live scrimmage) Blocking/checking (if applicable): - Can initiate age-appropriate checking against held pad - Progress to age-appropriate blocking/ body checking per hockey association guidelines
Phase 5 >60 minutes **Full pads**	Full contact practice participation	Full contact practice participation	Full contact practice participation

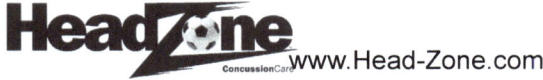
www.Head-Zone.com

LACROSSE

If headache, dizziness, or any other symptoms occur during any Phase, STOP exercising,
wait <u>24 hours</u>, and then resume activity at the <u>previous</u> symptom-free Phase/Day.
NOTE: Protective equipment should be worn when warranted

Exertion Phase	Cardio	Balance/Strength	Sports Drills
Phase 1 At least 15-20 minutes	<ul><li>Walking outside</li><li>Treadmill walking</li><li>Stationary bike</li><li>Arm Bike</li></ul>	<ul><li>Single leg balance</li><li>Tandem balance (one foot in front of the other)</li><li>Neck exercises (see handout)</li></ul>	<ul><li>Light stretching with team or in P.E class</li><li>May <u>walk</u> around gym, track, field in P.E. class</li></ul>
Phase 2 20 - 30 minutes	<ul><li>Walking (speed walk, walk uphill)</li><li>Elliptical</li><li>Stairmaster</li><li>Swim with kickboard</li><li>Light jump rope</li><li>Light jogging</li></ul>	<ul><li>Core exercises without head movement (ex. planks, leg lifts, etc.)</li><li>Body-weight exercises 1x10 (stationary lunges, squats, step-ups, push-ups, triceps dips, etc.)</li><li>Yoga and Pilates class (limit head movement)</li><li>Continue balance exercises</li></ul>	<ul><li>Activities with NO risk of collision or contact</li><li>NO activities with multiple balls flying through the air</li></ul>Examples:<ul><li>Light throw and catch/cradle with lacrosse stick</li><li>Stationary, low-intensity shooting</li></ul>
Phase 3 30 – 40 minutes Yellow (or contrast color) jersey should be worn to indicate NO contact Full pads/equipment	<ul><li>Maximize aerobic activity</li><li>Include running & sprinting</li><li>Accelerate to full speed with change of directions (cuts)</li></ul>	<ul><li>Core exercises w/head movement (ex. bicycle crunches, Russian twists, plank with head rotation)</li><li>Low-weight, high-repetition exercises 3x10 (ex. single-leg squats, walking lunges, 3-way lunges, bicep curls, bench press, etc.)</li><li>Dynamic warm-up (jogging, high knees, butt kicks, lunges, hip rotations etc.)</li><li>Jumping/impact exercises (squat jumps, jumping jacks, wall ball passes, progress to box jumps)</li><li>Balance exercises (ex. single-leg balance with forward reach to floor)</li></ul>	**Phase 3 is NON-CONTACT; emphasize stick/ball handling drills without an opponent**<ul><li>Agility/ladder drills</li><li>Cradle/catch drills</li><li>Ground ball drills</li><li>Shooting drills (shooting on the run, give & go, etc.)</li><li>Passing drills (waterfall drill pinwheel drill, etc.)</li></ul>Goalies:<ul><li>Non-competitive goalie drills with coach including agility drills with tennis ball, progressing to in goal shots (no rapid fire & no live scrimmage shots)</li><li>Practice 'clearing'</li><li>Work on movement required when ball is behind goal, in front of goal, and being passed from side to side</li></ul>
Phase 4 40 – 60 minutes Full pads/equipment	<ul><li>Continue Phase 3 Cardio, increasing in duration</li></ul>	<ul><li>Advanced core exercises (burpees, mountain climbers, etc.)</li><li>Can perform higher-weight, low-repetition exercises 4x3 (ex. Olympic Lifts, etc.)</li><li>Continue balance exercises</li></ul>	**Incorporate drills with an opponent (no live scrimmaging)**<ul><li>Pick & roll, 1 v 1, progressing to 2 v 2, etc.</li><li>Can initiate appropriate checking in drills</li><li>Goalies may take shots from players (non-competitive)</li></ul>
Phase 5 >60 minutes	Full contact practice participation	Full contact practice participation	Full contact practice participation

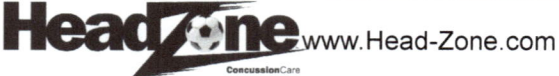
www.Head-Zone.com

MARTIAL ARTS

If headache, dizziness, or any other symptoms occur during any phase, STOP exercising.
Wait 24 hours, and then resume activity at the previous symptom-free Phase/Day

Exertion Phase	Cardio	Balance/Strength	Sports Drills
Phase 1 At least 15-20 minutes	▪ Walking outside ▪ Treadmill walking ▪ Stationary bike ▪ Arm Bike	▪ Single leg balance ▪ Tandem balance (one foot in front of the other) ▪ Neck exercises (see handout)	▪ Light stretching with team or in P.E class ▪ May <u>walk</u> around gym, track, field in P.E. class
Phase 2 20 - 30 minutes	▪ Walking (speed walk, walk uphill) ▪ Elliptical ▪ Stairmaster ▪ Swim with kickboard ▪ Light jump rope ▪ Light jogging	▪ Core exercises without head movement (ex. planks, leg lifts, etc.) ▪ Body-weight exercises 1x10 (stationary lunges, squats, step-ups, push-ups, triceps dips, etc.) ▪ Yoga and Pilates class (limit head movement) ▪ Continue balance exercises	▪ Activities with NO risk of collision or contact ▪ NO activities with multiple balls flying through the air Examples: ▪ Stationary, low-intensity punch ▪ Low-level forms
Phase 3 30 – 40 minutes	▪ Maximize aerobic activity ▪ Include running & sprinting ▪ Accelerate to full speed with change of directions (cuts)	▪ Core exercises w/head movement (ex. bicycle crunches, Russian twists, plank with head rotation) ▪ Low-weight, high-repetition exercises 3x10 (ex. single-leg squats, walking lunges, 3-way lunges, bicep curls, bench press, etc.) ▪ Dynamic warm-up (jogging, high knees, butt kicks, lunges, hip rotations etc.) ▪ Jumping/impact exercises (squat jumps, jumping jacks, wall ball passes, progress to box jumps) ▪ Balance exercises (ex. single-leg balance with forward reach to floor)	All non-contact drills ▪ High-intensity kicks and punches in air ▪ High-level forms ▪ Practice rolls
Phase 4 40 – 60 minutes	▪ Continue Phase 3 Cardio, increasing in duration	▪ Advanced core exercises (burpees, mountain climbers, etc.) ▪ Can perform higher-weight, low-repetition exercises 4x3 ▪ Continue balance exercises	▪ No Sparring ▪ No throwing
Phase 5 >60 minutes	Full contact practice participation	Full contact practice participation	Full contact practice participation

HeadZone
www.Head-Zone.com

RESISTANCE TRAINING & METABOLIC CONDITIONING

If headache, dizziness, or any other symptoms occur during any Phase, STOP exercising, wait <u>24 hours</u>, and then resume activity at the <u>previous</u> symptom-free Phase/Day.
NOTE: Protective equipment should be worn when warranted (e.g., helmet, mouth guard, pads)

Exertion Phase	Cardio	Balance/Strength
Phase 1 At least 15-20 minutes	<ul><li>Walking outside</li><li>Treadmill walking</li><li>Stationary bike</li><li>Arm Bike</li></ul>	<ul><li>Single leg balance</li><li>Tandem balance (one foot in front of the other)</li><li>Neck exercises (see handout)</li></ul>
Phase 2 20 – 30 minutes	<ul><li>Walking (speed walk, walk uphill)</li><li>Elliptical</li><li>Stairmaster</li><li>Light jump rope</li><li>Light jogging</li></ul>	<ul><li>Core exercises without head movement (ex. planks, leg lifts, etc.)</li><li>Body-weight exercises 1 x10<ul><li>Stationary lunges</li><li>Squats</li><li>Step-ups</li><li>Push-ups</li><li>Triceps dips, etc.</li></ul></li><li>Yoga and Pilates class (limit head movement)</li><li>Continue balance exercises (above)</li></ul>
Phase 3 30 – 40 minutes	<ul><li>Running & sprinting</li><li>Accelerate to full speed with change of directions</li><li>Emphasize quick acceleration and deceleration</li><li>Example: 10 minute walk/jog on treadmill, 10 minutes on the elliptical, 10 minutes on a stationary bike</li></ul>	Continue above exercises; Add **2 x 10** of the following<ul><li>Core exercises w/head movement (ex. bicycle crunches, Russian twists, plank with head rotation, cable twists, supine bridge, etc.)</li></ul>Resistance training exercises; 3-4 sets x 10-15 repetitions; <30 second rest between sets<ul><li>Single-leg squats, walking lunges, 3-way lunges, bicep curls, dumbbell bench press, seated rows, kettlebell swings, pull-ups etc.</li></ul>60%-70% of 1 rep. max:_____<ul><li>Dynamic warm-up (jogging, high knees, butt kicks, lunges, hip rotations etc.</li><li>Jumping/impact exercises (squat jumps, jumping jacks, wall ball passes, progress to box jumps</li><li>Balance exercises (ex. single-leg balance with forward reach to floor)</li></ul>
Phase 4 40 – 60 minutes	<ul><li>Continue Phase 3 cardio, increasing in intensity and duration</li><li>Example for cardio intervals: treadmill – 20 second fast-paced jog, 10 second walk (repeat 8-10 times)</li></ul>	Advanced core exercises<ul><li>Burpees, mountain climbers, roll-outs, weighted dead-bug, stir the pot, body saw, single arm farmers carry, pallof press, etc.</li></ul>Higher-weight, low-repetition exercises 1-3 sets x 8-12 repetitions; 30s – 1.5 min. rest between setsSift, dumbbell split squat, lat pulldown, bent over row, bench press, shoulder press 67%-80% of 1 rep. max:_____<ul><li>Continue balance exercises (above)</li></ul>
Phase 5 >60 minutes	Full participation	Full session of resistance training and metabolic conditioning

HeadZone www.Head-Zone.com

ROWING

If headache, dizziness, or any other symptoms occur during any Phase, STOP exercising, wait <u>24 hours</u>, and then resume activity at the <u>previous</u> symptom-free Phase/Day.

Exertion Phase	Cardio	Balance/strength	Sports Drills
Phase 1 At least 15-20 minutes	- Walking outside - Treadmill walking - Stationary bike - Arm Bike	- Single leg balance - Tandem balance (one foot in front of the other) - Neck exercises (see handout)	- Light stretching with team or in P.E class - May <u>walk</u> around gym, track, field in P.E. class
Phase 2 20 - 30 minutes	- Walking (speed walk, walk uphill) - Elliptical - Stairmaster - Swim with kickboard - Light jump rope - Light jogging	- Core exercises without head movement (ex. planks, leg lifts, etc.) - Body-weight exercises 1x10 (stationary lunges, squats, step-ups, push-ups, triceps dips, etc.) - Yoga and Pilates class (limit head movement) - Continue balance exercises	- Activities with NO risk of collision or contact - NO activities with multiple balls flying through the air Examples: - Low-intensity erg (indoor rowing machine)
Phase 3 30 – 40 minutes	- Running & sprinting - Accelerate to full speed with change of directions (cuts) - Emphasize quick acceleration and deceleration	- Core exercises w/head movement (ex. bicycle crunches, Russian twists, plank with head rotation) - Low-weight, high-repetition exercises 3x10 (ex. single-leg squats, walking lunges, 3-way lunges, bicep curls, bench press, etc.) - Dynamic warm-up (jogging, high skips, side shuffles, jumping jacks, high knees, butt kicks, etc.) - Jumping/impact exercises (squat jumps, jumping jacks, wall ball passes, progress to box jumps) - Balance exercises (ex. single-leg balance with forward reach to floor)	- Progress erg intensity and duration prior to going out on the water - Emphasize strength training (upper and lower body) - May initiate on-water rowing in a beginner, single-person boat
Phase 4 40 – 60 minutes	- Continue Phase 3 cardio, increasing intensity and duration	- Advanced core exercises (burpees, mountain climbers, etc.) - Can incorporate higher-weight, low-repetition exercises 4x3 (ex. Olympic Lifts, etc.) - Continue balance exercises	- Progress to moderate-intensity rowing with multiple rowers (i.e. in a two, four, etc. person boat)
Phase 5 >60 minutes	Full practice participation	Full practice participation	Full practice participation

HeadZone
www.Head-Zone.com

RUGBY

If headache, dizziness, or any other symptoms occur during any Phase, STOP exercising, wait <u>24 hours</u>, and then resume activity at the <u>previous</u> symptom-free Phase/Day.

Exertion Phase	Cardio	Balance/Strength	Sports Drills
Phase 1 At least 15-20 minutes	- Walking outside - Treadmill walking - Stationary bike - Arm Bike	- Single leg balance - Tandem balance (one foot in front of the other) - Neck exercises (see handout)	- Light stretching with team or in P.E class - May <u>walk</u> around gym, track, field in P.E. class
Phase 2 20 - 30 minutes	- Walking (speed walk, walk uphill) - Elliptical - Stairmaster - Swim with kickboard - Light jump rope - Light jogging	- Core exercises without head movement (ex. planks, leg lifts, etc.) - Body-weight exercises 1x10 (stationary lunges, squats, step-ups, push-ups, triceps dips, etc.) - Yoga and Pilates class (limit head movement) - Continue balance exercises	- Activities with NO risk of collision or contact - NO activities with multiple balls flying through the air Examples: - Low-intensity kicks - Low-intensity short passes
Phase 3 30 – 40 minutes Yellow (or contrast color) jersey should be worn to indicate NO contact	- Running & sprinting - Accelerate to full speed with change of directions (cuts) - Emphasize quick acceleration and deceleration	- Core exercises w/head movement (ex. bicycle crunches, Russian twists, plank with head rotation) - Low-weight, high-repetition exercises 3x10 (ex. single-leg squats, walking lunges, 3- way lunges, bicep curls, bench press, etc.) - Dynamic warm-up (jogging, high knees, butt kicks, lunges, hip rotations etc.) - Jumping/impact exercises (squat jumps, jumping jacks, wall ball passes, progress to box jumps) - Balance exercises (ex. single-leg balance with forward reach to floor)	**Phase 3 is NON-CONTACT** Only <u>light hand-touch contact</u> in drills with NO chance of collision with another player Examples: - Agility/ladder drills - Footwork drills -swerve, spin and offload the ball (mimic avoiding tackles and keeping the ball moving) - Passing/handling drills with teammates - Progress passing length and intensity
Phase 4 40 – 60 minutes	- Continue Phase 3 Cardio, increasing intensity and duration	- Advanced core exercises (burpees, mountain climbers, etc.) - Higher-weight, low-repetition exercises 4x3 (ex. Olympic Lifts, etc.) - Continue balance exercises	Can incorporate body contact in drills (no live scrimmage) - Begin tackling a dummy with a slow motion tackle from one knee; progress to tackling from standing with dummy - Progress to tackling 1 v 1, 2 v 2, 2 v 1 etc. - Practice falling correctly and tackling in a ruck - Scrum drills with dummy - Practice mauling by ripping the ball out, 1 v 1 then incorporating other players - Line-out
Phase 5 >60 minutes	Full contact practice participation	Full contact practice participation	Full contact practice participation

HeadZone www.Head-Zone.com

SKIING & SNOWBOARDING

If headache, dizziness, or any other symptoms occur during any Phase, STOP exercising, wait <u>24 hours</u>, and then resume activity at the <u>previous</u> symptom-free Phase/Day.

NOTE: Protective equipment should be worn when warranted (ex. helmet)

Exertion Phase	Cardio	Balance/Strength	Sports Drills
Phase 1 At least 15-20 minutes	- Walking outside - Treadmill walking - Stationary bike - Arm Bike	- Single leg balance - Tandem balance (one foot in front of the other) - Neck exercises (see handout)	- Light stretching with team or in P.E class - May <u>walk</u> around gym, track, field in P.E. class
Phase 2 20 - 30 minutes	- Walking (speed walk, walk uphill) - Elliptical - Stairmaster - Swim with kickboard - Light jump rope - Light jogging	- Core exercises without head movement (ex. planks, leg lifts, etc.) - Body-weight exercises 1x10 (stationary lunges, squats, step-ups, push-ups, triceps dips, etc.) - Yoga and Pilates class (limit head movement) - Continue balance exercises	- Activities with NO risk of collision or contact - NO activities with multiple balls flying through the air - No skiing or snowboarding Examples: - Slide board and Pro-fitter in PT - Balance board
Phase 3 30 – 40 minutes	- Maximize aerobic activity - Include running & sprinting - Accelerate to full speed with change of directions (cuts)	- Core exercises w/head movement (ex. bicycle crunches, Russian twists, plank with head rotation) - Low-weight, high-repetition exercises 3x10 (ex. single-leg squats, walking lunges, 3- way lunges, bicep curls, bench press, etc.) - Dynamic warm-up (jogging, high knees, butt kicks, lunges, hip rotations etc.) - Jumping/impact exercises (squat jumps, jumping jacks, wall ball passes, progress to box jumps) - Balance exercises (ex. single-leg balance with forward reach to floor)	- Begin with low-intensity skiing/ riding on small to medium sized hills (green or blue) - Avoid crowded hills and icy conditions - Begin skiing/snowboarding at 'off –hours' to avoid risk of collision with other skiers/snowboarders - Progress to big hills (black, double black diamond) and higher-intensity skiing/riding - No moguls - No flips/tricks BE AWARE OF YOUR SURROUNDINGS AT ALL TIMES!
Phase 4 40 – 60 minutes	- Continue Phase 3 Cardio, increasing in duration	- Advanced core exercises (burpees, mountain climbers, etc.) - Can incorporate higher-weight, low-repetition exercises - Continue balance exercises	- Can begin tricks; start with small jumps and small boxes - Progress to medium sized jumps and medium sized boxes - Progress to rails - No flips - Low intensity moguls progressing to higher intensity moguls
Phase 5 >60 minutes	Full participation in practice/lessons	Full participation in practice/lessons	Full participation in practice/lessons -Can incorporate flips

www.Head-Zone.com

SOCCER

If headache, dizziness, or any other symptoms occur during any Phase, STOP exercising, wait <u>24 hours</u>, and then resume activity at the <u>previous</u> symptom-free Phase/Day.

Exertion Phase	Cardio	Balance/Strength	Sports Drills
Phase 1 At least 15-20 minutes	- Walking outside - Treadmill walking - Stationary bike - Arm Bike	- Single leg balance - Tandem balance (one foot in front of the other) - Neck exercises (see handout)	- Light stretching with team or in P.E class - May <u>walk</u> around gym, track, field in P.E. class
Phase 2 20 - 30 minutes	- Walking (speed walk, walk uphill) - Elliptical - Stairmaster - Swim with kickboard - Light jump rope - Light jogging	- Core exercises without head movement (ex. planks, leg lifts, etc.) - Body-weight exercises 1x10 (stationary lunges, squats, step-ups, push-ups, triceps dips, etc.) - Yoga and Pilates class (limit head movement) - Continue balance exercises	- Activities with NO risk of collision or contact - NO activities with multiple balls flying through the air Examples: - Soccer footwork - Low-intensity passing and shooting
Phase 3 30 – 40 minutes **Yellow (or contrast color) jersey should be worn to indicate NO contact**	- Running & sprinting - Accelerate to full speed with change of directions (cuts) - Emphasize quick acceleration and deceleration	- Core exercises w/head movement (ex. bicycle crunches, Russian twists, plank with head rotation) - Low-weight, high-repetition exercises 3x10 (ex. single-leg squats, walking lunges, 3- way lunges, bicep curls, bench press, etc.) - Dynamic warm-up (jogging, high knees, butt kicks, lunges, hip rotations etc.) - Jumping/impact exercises (squat jumps, jumping jacks, wall ball passes, progress to box jumps) - Balance exercises (ex. single-leg balance with forward reach to floor)	All drills with **NO OPPONENT** and **NO** chance of collision with another player **NO heading** - Warm-up drills - Agility/Ladder drills - Ball skills - Shooting/chipping drills - Passing drills (practice long and short passes) Goal-keeper: - Non-competitive goalie drills (with coach) including agility drills with tennis ball, progressing to in goal catches (no rapid fire & no live scrimmage shots) - Punts - Distribution drills
Phase 4 40 – 60 minutes	- Continue Phase 3 cardio, increasing in intensity and duration	- Advanced core exercises (burpees, mountain climbers, etc.) - Can perform higher-weight, low-repetition exercises 4x3 (ex. Olympic Lifts, etc.) - Continue balance exercises	- Incorporate drills with an opponent (no live scrimmaging) -**NO heading** - 1 v1, 2 v 2, etc. opponent drills Goal-keeper: - Dives from knees (progress to standing) - May catch shots from players (non-competitive)
Phase 5 >60 minutes	Full contact practice participation	Full contact practice participation	Full contact practice participation *Heading not recommended*

HeadZone www.Head-Zone.com

SQUASH

If headache, dizziness, or any other symptoms occur during any Phase, STOP exercising, wait <u>24 hours</u>, and then resume activity at the <u>previous</u> symptom-free Phase/Day.

Exertion Phase	Cardio	Balance/strength	Sports Drills
Phase 1 At least 15-20 minutes	- Walking outside - Treadmill walking - Stationary bike - Arm Bike	- Single leg balance - Tandem balance (one foot in front of the other) - Neck exercises (see handout)	- Light stretching with team or in P.E class - May <u>walk</u> around gym, track, field in P.E. class
Phase 2 20 - 30 minutes	- Walking (speed walk, walk uphill) - Elliptical - Stairmaster - Swim with kickboard - Light jump rope - Light jogging	- Core exercises without head movement (ex. planks, leg lifts, etc.) - Body-weight exercises 1x10 (stationary lunges, squats, step-ups, push-ups, triceps dips, etc.) - Yoga and Pilates class (limit head movement) - Continue balance exercises	- Activities with NO risk of collision or contact - NO activities with multiple balls flying through the air Examples: - Bounce a tennis ball against a wall - Progress to low-intensity forehand and backhand swings with ball
Phase 3 30 – 40 minutes	- Running & sprinting - Accelerate to full speed with change of directions (cuts) - Emphasize quick acceleration and deceleration	- Core exercises w/head movement (ex. bicycle crunches, Russian twists, plank with head rotation) - Low-weight, high-repetition exercises 3x10 (ex. single-leg squats, walking lunges, 3-way lunges, bicep curls, bench press, etc.) - Dynamic warm-up (jogging, high skips, side shuffles, jumping jacks, high knees, butt kicks, etc.) - Jumping/impact exercises (squat jumps, jumping jacks, wall ball passes, progress to box jumps) - Balance exercises (ex. single-leg balance with forward reach to floor)	- Serving: start with low-intensity serves working on form; and progress in intensity - Footwork drills (ex. run to the wall and back-peddle) - Moderate intensity volley with yourself (non-competitive)
Phase 4 40 – 60 minutes	- Continue Phase 3 cardio, increasing in duration	- Advanced core exercises (burpees, mountain climbers, etc.) - Can incorporate higher-weight, low-repetition exercises 4x3 (ex. Olympic Lifts, etc.) - Continue balance exercises	- Progress to higher intensity volleying with teammate then competitive play - Can play doubles (start in back position, progress to front position)
Phase 5 >60 minutes	Full practice participation	Full practice participation	Full practice participation

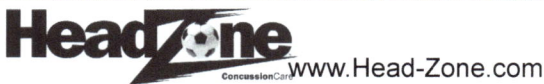
www.Head-Zone.com

SWIMMING

If headache, dizziness, or any other symptoms occur during any phase, STOP exercising.
Wait 24 hours, and then resume activity at the previous symptom-free Phase/Day.

Exertion Phase	Cardio	Balance/Strength	Sports Drills
Phase 1 At least 15-20 minutes	- Walking outside - Treadmill walking - Stationary bike - Arm Bike	- Single leg balance (3 x 30 sec) - Tandem balance (one foot in front of the other 2 x 15 sec) - Neck exercises (see handout)	- Light stretching with team or in P.E class - May <u>walk</u> around gym, track, field in P.E. class
Phase 2 20-30 minutes	- Elliptical - Stationary bike - Stair master - Light jogging - Light jump rope	- Core exercises without head movement (ex. planks, leg lifts, etc.) - Body-weight exercises 1x10 (stationary lunges, squats, step-ups, push-ups, triceps dips, etc.) - Yoga and Pilates class (limit head movement) - Continue balance exercises	- Activities with NO risk of collision or contact. - NO activities with multiple balls flying through the air Examples: - Swimming with kickboard - Low-intensity swimming underwater
Phase 3 30-40 minutes	- Running & sprinting - Accelerate to full speed with change of directions (cuts) - Emphasize quick acceleration and deceleration	- Core exercises w/head movement (ex. bicycle crunches, Russian twists, plank with head rotation) - Low-weight, high-repetition exercises 3x10 (ex. single-leg squats, walking lunges, 3-way lunges, bicep curls, bench press, etc.) - Dynamic warm-up (jogging, high skips, side shuffles, jumping jacks, high knees, butt kicks, etc.) - Jumping/impact exercises (squat jumps, jumping jacks, wall ball passes, progress to box jumps) - Balance exercises (ex. single-leg balance with forward reach to floor)	- No diving - No flip turns - Forward and backward rolls/flips while in the water - <u>Must swim in your own lane</u> (no risk of being kicked) - Begin low-intensity breast stroke and side stroke increasing in intensity - Must be able to tolerate exercise with head movement, then start low-intensity freestyle (progress in intensity) - Make sure flags are up before starting backstroke; swim back stroke progressing to wall touch - Begin swimming 50 m, progressing to 100m, etc. - No medley (individual or relay)
Phase 4 40-60 minutes	- Continue Phase 3 cardio, increasing intensity and duration	- Advanced core exercises (burpees, mountain climbers, etc.) - Can incorporate higher-weight, low-repetition exercises 4x3 (ex. Olympic Lifts, etc.) - Continue balance exercises	- Dive from side of pool - Add flip turns in pool - Begin butterfly - Increase stroke intensity and duration to race speed/duration - Initiate individual medley, progressing to medley relay
Phase 5 > 60 minutes	Full practice participation	Full practice participation	Full practice participation; diving off block; swim in lane with other swimmers

HeadZone www.Head-Zone.com

TENNIS

If headache, dizziness, or any other symptoms occur during any Phase, STOP exercising, wait <u>24 hours</u>, and then resume activity at the <u>previous</u> symptom-free Phase/Day.

Exertion Phase	Cardio	Balance/strength	Sports Drills
Phase 1 At least 15-20 minutes	- Walking outside - Treadmill walking - Stationary bike - Arm Bike	- Single leg balance - Tandem balance (one foot in front of the other) - Neck exercises (see handout)	- Light stretching with team or in P.E class - May <u>walk</u> around gym, track, field in P.E. class

Phase 2
 	
20 - 30 minutes
	- Walking (speed walk, walk uphill)
	- Elliptical
	- Stairmaster
	- Swim with kickboard
	- Light jump rope
	- Light jogging
		- Core exercises without head movement (ex. planks, leg lifts, etc.)
		- Body-weight exercises 1x10 (stationary lunges, squats, step-ups, push-ups, triceps dips, etc.)
		- Yoga and Pilates class (limit head movement)
		- Continue balance exercises
			- Activities with NO risk of collision or contact
			- NO activities with multiple balls flying through the air
			- Examples:
			  - Bounce a tennis ball against a wall
			  - Progress to low-intensity forehand and backhand swings with ball

Phase 3 30 – 40 minutes	- Running & sprinting - Accelerate to full speed with change of directions (cuts) - Emphasize quick acceleration and deceleration	- Core exercises w/head movement (ex. bicycle crunches, Russian twists, plank with head rotation) - Low-weight, high-repetition exercises 3x10 (ex. single-leg squats, walking lunges, 3-way lunges, bicep curls, bench press, etc.) - Dynamic warm-up (jogging, high skips, side shuffles, jumping jacks, high knees, butt kicks, etc.) - Jumping/impact exercises (squat jumps, jumping jacks, wall ball passes, progress to box jumps) - Balance exercises (ex. single-leg balance with forward reach to floor)	- Serving: start with low-intensity serves working on form; and progress in intensity - Footwork drills (ex. run to the net and back-peddle) - Moderate intensity volley with coach (non-competitive)
Phase 4 40 – 60 minutes	- Continue Phase 3 cardio, increasing in duration	- Advanced core exercises (burpees, mountain climbers, etc.) - Can incorporate higher-weight, low-repetition exercises 4x3 (ex. Olympic Lifts, etc.) - Continue balance exercises	- Progress to higher intensity volleying with teammate then competitive play - Can play doubles (start in back position, progress to front position)
Phase 5 >60 minutes	Full practice participation	Full practice participation	Full practice participation

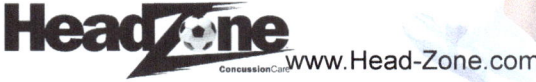
www.Head-Zone.com

TOUCH SPARRING

If headache, dizziness, or any other symptoms occur during any Phase, STOP exercising, wait <u>24 hours</u>, and then resume activity at the <u>previous</u> symptom-free Phase/Day.

Exertion Phase	Cardio	Balance/Strength	Sports Drills
Phase 1 At least 15-20 minutes	▪ Walking outside ▪ Treadmill walking ▪ Stationary bike ▪ Arm Bike	▪ Single leg balance ▪ Tandem balance (one foot in front of the other) ▪ Neck exercises (see handout)	▪ Light stretching with team or in P.E class ▪ May <u>walk</u> around gym, track, field in P.E. class
Phase 2 20 - 30 minutes	▪ Walking (speed walk, walk uphill) ▪ Elliptical ▪ Stairmaster ▪ Swim with kickboard ▪ Light jump rope ▪ Light jogging	▪ Core exercises without head movement (ex. planks, leg lifts, etc.) ▪ Body-weight exercises 1x10 (stationary lunges, squats, step-ups, push-ups, triceps dips, etc.) ▪ Yoga and Pilates class (limit head movement) ▪ Continue balance exercises	▪ Activities with NO risk of collision or contact ▪ NO activities with multiple balls flying through the air
Phase 3 30 – 40 minutes	▪ Maximize aerobic activity ▪ Include running & sprinting ▪ Accelerate to full speed with change of directions (cuts)	▪ Core exercises w/head movement (ex. bicycle crunches, Russian twists, plank with head rotation) ▪ Low-weight, high-repetition exercises 3x10 (ex. single-leg squats, walking lunges, 3-way lunges, bicep curls, bench press, etc.) ▪ Dynamic warm-up (jogging, high knees, butt kicks, lunges, hip rotations, backward sprint, etc.) ▪ Jumping/impact exercises (squat jumps, jumping jacks, wall ball passes, progress to box jumps) ▪ Balance exercises (ex. single-leg balance with forward reach to floor)	▪ Footwork without an opponent ▪ Shadow boxing ▪ Moderate intensity pad work with coach ▪ Moderate intensity speedbag work ▪ Moderate to heavy intensity bag work NO LIVE SPARRING!
Phase 4 40 – 60 minutes	▪ Continue Phase 3 Cardio, increasing in duration	▪ Advanced core exercises (burpees, mountain climbers, etc.) ▪ Higher-weight, low-repetition exercises 4x3 (ex. Olympic Lifts, etc.) ▪ Continue balance exercises	▪ Footwork with an opponent (no gloves) ▪ Heavy pad work with coach ▪ High intensity speedbag work ▪ High intensity heavy bag work ▪ NO LIVE SPARRING!
Phase 5 >60 minutes	Full touch sparring	Full touch sparring	Full touch sparring

HeadZone www.Head-Zone.com

TRACK & FIELD

If headache, dizziness, or any other symptoms occur during any Phase, STOP exercising, wait <u>24 hours</u>, and then resume activity at the <u>previous</u> symptom-free Phase/Day.

Exertion Phase	Cardio	Balance/strength	Sports Drills
Phase 1 At least 15-20 minutes	<ul><li>Walking outside</li><li>Treadmill walking</li><li>Stationary bike</li><li>Arm Bike</li></ul>	<ul><li>Single leg balance</li><li>Tandem balance (one foot in front of the other)</li><li>Neck exercises (see handout)</li></ul>	<ul><li>Light stretching with team or in P.E class</li><li>May <u>walk</u> around gym, track, field in P.E. class</li></ul>
Phase 2 20 - 30 minutes	<ul><li>Walking (speed walk, walk uphill)</li><li>Elliptical</li><li>Stairmaster</li><li>Swim with kickboard</li><li>Light jump rope</li><li>Light jogging</li></ul>	<ul><li>Core exercises without head movement (ex. planks, leg lifts, etc.)</li><li>Body-weight exercises 1x10 (stationary lunges, squats, step-ups, push-ups, triceps dips, etc.)</li><li>Yoga and Pilates class (limit head movement)</li><li>Continue balance exercises</li></ul>	<ul><li>Activities with NO risk of collision or contact</li><li>NO activities with multiple balls flying through the air</li></ul>Examples:<ul><li>Jog around track</li><li>Slow throwing technique (half-speed or slower); no spins</li></ul>
Phase 3 30 – 40 minutes	<ul><li>Running & sprinting</li><li>Accelerate to full speed with change of directions (cuts)</li><li>Emphasize quick acceleration and deceleration</li></ul>	<ul><li>Core exercises w/head movement (ex. bicycle crunches, Russian twists, plank with head rotation)</li><li>Low-weight, high-repetition exercises 3x10 (ex. single-leg squats, walking lunges, 3-way lunges, bicep curls, bench press, etc.)</li><li>Dynamic warm-up (jogging, high skips, side shuffles, jumping jacks, high knees, butt kicks, etc.)</li><li>Jumping/impact exercises (squat jumps, jumping jacks, wall ball passes, progress to box jumps)</li><li>Balance exercises (ex. single-leg balance with forward reach to floor)</li></ul>	<ul><li><u>Sprinters</u>: Focus on quick start technique; sprint short distances, progress to competition intensity/duration</li><li><u>Horizontal jumpers</u>: begin with low-intensity jumps; progress in intensity</li><li><u>High jumpers</u>: begin with low-intensity/height jumps focusing on proper landing technique</li><li><u>Pole vault</u>: jog and push pole overhead; progress to low-level pole vault with landing on feet</li><li><u>Throwers</u>: advance stationary throwing intensity and progress to spins</li><li><u>Hurdles/steeple jump</u>: No hurdles or steeple jump; place emphasis on increasing running speed and duration</li></ul>
Phase 4 40 – 60 minutes	<ul><li>Continue Phase 3 Cardio, increasing intensity and duration</li></ul>	<ul><li>Advanced core exercises (burpees, mountain climbers, etc.)</li><li>Can incorporate higher-weight, low-repetition exercises 4x3 (ex. Olympic Lifts, etc.)</li><li>Continue balance exercises</li></ul>	<ul><li><u>High jumpers</u>: progress height of jumps</li><li><u>Pole vault</u>: Low-level landing on back, progressing to higher-level</li><li><u>Hurdles/steeple jump</u>: practice with low-level hurdle; progress to full competition level</li></ul>
Phase 5 >60 minutes	Full practice participation	Full practice participation	Full practice participation

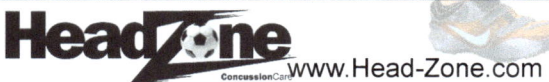

VOLLEYBALL

If headache, dizziness, or any other symptoms occur during any Phase, STOP exercising, wait <u>24 hours</u>, and then resume activity at the <u>previous</u> symptom-free Phase/Day.
NOTE: Protective equipment should be worn when warranted (ex. knee pads)

Exertion Phase	Cardio	Balance/Strength	Sports Drills
Phase 1 At least 15-20 minutes	<ul><li>Walking outside Tread-mill walking</li><li>Stationary bike</li><li>Arm Bike</li></ul>	<ul><li>Single leg balance</li><li>Tandem balance (one foot in front of the other)</li><li>Neck exercises (see handout)</li></ul>	<ul><li>Light stretching with team or in P.E class</li><li>May <u>walk</u> around gym, track, field in P.E. class</li></ul>
Phase 2 20 - 30 minutes	<ul><li>Walking (speed walk, walk uphill)</li><li>Elliptical</li><li>Stairmaster</li><li>Swim with kickboard</li><li>Light jump rope</li><li>Light jogging</li></ul>	<ul><li>Core exercises without head movement (ex. planks, leg lifts, etc.)</li><li>Body-weight exercises 1x10 (stationary lunges, squats, step-ups, push-ups, triceps dips, etc.)</li><li>Yoga and Pilates class (limit head movement)</li><li>Continue balance exercises</li></ul>	<ul><li>Activities with NO risk of collision or contact</li><li>NO activities with multiple balls flying through the air</li></ul>Examples:<ul><li>Stationary, low-intensity serving</li><li>Low-intensity hitting, passing, setting</li></ul>
Phase 3 30 – 40 minutes	<ul><li>Running & sprinting</li><li>Accelerate to full speed with change of directions (cuts)</li><li>Emphasize quick acceleration and deceleration</li></ul>	<ul><li>Core exercises w/head movement (ex. bicycle crunches, Russian twists, plank with head rotation)</li><li>Low-weight, high-repetition exercises 3x10 (ex. single-leg squats, walking lunges, 3-way lunges, bicep curls, bench press, etc.)</li><li>Dynamic warm-up (jogging, high knees, butt kicks, lunges, hip rotations etc.)</li><li>Jumping/impact exercises (squat jumps, jumping jacks, wall ball passes, progress to box jumps)</li><li>Balance exercises (ex. single-leg balance with forward reach to floor)</li></ul>	<ul><li>Activities with NO risk of collision or contact</li><li>NO activities with multiple balls flying through the air</li><li>Agility/ladder drills</li><li>Practice serving; progressing to full intensity</li><li>Hitting, setting, passing drills with teammates</li><li>Practice diving for ball from knees</li></ul>
Phase 4 40 – 60 minutes	<ul><li>Continue Phase 3 Cardio, increasing intensity and duration</li></ul>	<ul><li>Advanced core exercises (burpees, mountain climbers, etc.)</li><li>Can incorporate higher-weight, low-repetition exercises</li><li>Continue balance exercises</li></ul>	<ul><li>No live scrimmage</li><li>Full intensity drills with teammates (Ex. volley pass, pass & move, dig technique, defensive dig drills, pepper)</li><li>Progress to diving from standing</li></ul>
Phase 5 >60 minutes	Full practice participation	Full practice participation	Full practice participation

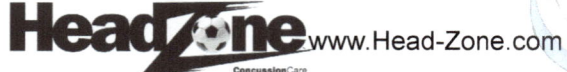

WRESTLING

If headache, dizziness, or any other symptoms occur during any Phase, STOP exercising, wait <u>24 hours</u>, and then resume activity at the <u>previous</u> symptom-free Phase/Day.

Exertion Phase	Cardio	Balance/Strength	Sports Drills
Phase 1 At least 15-20 minutes	- Walking outside - Treadmill walking - Stationary bike - Arm Bike	- Single leg balance - Tandem balance (one foot in front of the other) - Neck exercises (see handout)	- Light stretching with team or in P.E class - May <u>walk</u> around gym, track, field in P.E. class
Phase 2 20 - 30 minutes	- Walking (speed walk, walk uphill) - Elliptical - Stairmaster - Swim with kickboard - Light jump rope - Light jogging	- Core exercises without head movement (ex. planks, leg lifts, etc.) - Body-weight exercises 1x10 (stationary lunges, squats, step-ups, push-ups, triceps dips, etc.) - Yoga and Pilates class (limit head movement) - Continue balance exercises	- Activities with NO risk of collision or contact - NO activities with multiple balls flying through the air
Phase 3 30 – 40 minutes	- Running & sprinting - Accelerate to full speed with change of directions (cuts) - Emphasize quick acceleration and deceleration	- Core exercises w/head movement (ex. bicycle crunches, Russian twists, plank with head rotation) - Low-weight, high-repetition exercises 3x10 (ex. single-leg squats, walking lunges, 3- way lunges, bicep curls, bench press, etc.) - Dynamic warm-up (jogging, high knees, butt kicks, lunges, hip rotations, backward sprint, etc.) - Jumping/impact exercises (squat jumps, jumping jacks, wall ball passes, progress to box jumps) - Balance exercises (ex. single-leg balance with forward reach to floor)	**Phase 3 is NON-CONTACT** Only <u>light hand-touch contact</u> in wrestling drills Examples: - Agility/ladder drills - Crawls (Bear, army, duck crawls, etc.) - Sideways plank walk - Stance and motion - Scramble to stance - Mirror drill - Buddy Carry drills - Limbo level change

Phase 4
 	
40 – 60 minutes
	- Continue Phase 3 Cardio, increasing intensity and duration	- Advanced core exercises (burpees, mountain climbers, etc.)
		- Higher-weight, low-repetition exercises 4x3 (ex. Olympic Lifts, etc.)
		- Continue balance exercises
			Controlled contact wrestling drills (no live wrestling)
			- Advanced agility drills with body contact
			Examples:
			  -Shooting drills
			  -Stand-up returns
			  -Jolt drill
			  -Spin Drill
			- Practice situation wrestling

Phase 5 >60 minutes	Full contact practice participation	Full contact practice participation	Full contact practice participation (live wrestling at practice)

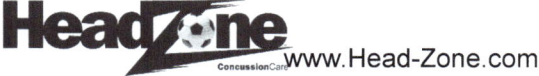